TEXT BOOK ON ABUSE OF ALCOHOL AND DRUGS

AJITHA NANCY RANI.R

PROFESSOR SREE BALAJI COLLEGE OF NURSING

RIGI PUBLICATION

TEXT BOOK ON ABUSE OF ALCOHOL AND DRUGS

By

AJITHA NANCY RANI.R

Copyright© AJITHA NANCY RANI.R 2022

Originally published in India

Edition: 1

ISBN: 978-93-91041-54-0

Published by RIGI PUBLICATION

777, Street no.9, Krishna Nagar Khanna-141401 (Punjab), India

Website: www.rigipublication.com

Email: info@rigipublication.com

Phone: +91-9357710014, +91-9465468291

ACKNOWLEDGEMENT

I would express a deep sense of gratitude to the almighty who is continuously giving the support and guidance required in all my deeds, and would like to express my gratitude to all who guided, advised and moulded this piece of work and provided information, without which I would never have completed this endeavour.

I owe a great deal of thanks to my teachers and friends who is the spirit of inspiration in taking up the project.

I extend my sincere thanks to the most respected and DR.V.Hemavathy, M.Sc (Nursing), M.A, M.Phil,Ph.D., Principal, Sree Balaji College of Nursing, for guiding me to uplift my professional career by her valuable and constant guidance throughout this study The reason for writing this book is to satisfy the B.SC NURSING, students and empower them in psychiatry.

As the result of changes in standards and challenges in psychiatric nursing, nurses should be trained toapply the basic concept and principles of psychiatic nursing in various settings.

This book is written in a simple text, easy to read and understand and precisely to answer their exam questions. For those who are interested in psychiatry they may read other comprehensive text books available.

I sincerely acknowledge my thanks to my beloved husband Mr T.Stephen Kishore, my children, Derrick Samuel Raj, Hannah Jerusha and my colleagues. I will appreciate the comments and suggestions for improving the book.

THE ABUSE OF ALCOHOL AND DRUGS

(Drug Addiction)

The term substance use disorder (DSM IV) is disorder due to psychoactive drug use and (ICD-10) is used to refer to conditions arising from the abuse of alcohol, psychoactive drugs, prescription and over the counter drugs (OTCdrugs) and other chemicals such as volatile solvents.Psychoactive substances are compounds that can alter a persons state of mind. Throughout history in all cultures, people have sought out substances that alter consciousness or mood.

SUBSTANCE USE DISORDER

Substance-related disorders are composed of two groups: the substance-use disorders dependence and abuse and the substance-induced disorders (intoxication, withdrawal, delirium, dementia, amnesia, psychosis, mood disorder, anxiety disorder, sexual dysfunction, and sleep disorders).To use wrongfully or in a harmful way. Improper treatment or conduct that may result in injury. The need is so strong as to generate distress (either physical or psychological) if left unfulfilled.

The commonly used and abused psychoactive substances can be grouped as follows:

1. Alcohol.
2. Illegal drugs.
- Opiates (E.g.). Heroin, Pethidine, Codeine, and Pentazocine.
- Stimulants (E.g) Cocaine, amphetamines, ecstasy.
- Hallucinogens (E.g) LS.

3. a) Others (Eg) Cannabis, caffeine, and nicotine.

b) PRESCRIPTION AND OTC DRUGS:

- Benzodiazepines.
- Barbiturates.
- Cough Syrup.
- Antihistamine.

4. Volatile Substances: Inhalants

- Glues, petrol, nail polish, adhesives, typing eraser etc.,
  Some common terminology in the substance use disorders.

ADDICTION:

Loss of control over drug use (including OH), typically manifested as compulsive seeking and taking of drugs despite abnormal consequences. Addiction requires repeated drug and exposure as well as a vulnerable brain. The term addiction has been replaced by drug dependence by the WHO.

HARMFUL USE:

(Abuse) refer to maladaptive patterns of substance use that impairs health in a broad sense.

DRUG DEPENDENCE (SUBSTANCE DEPENDECE)

It is characterized by a typical drug seeking behaviour which becomes the most important priority in person's life in spite of the psychosocial impairment caused by the use of the substance, and the development of tolerance or withdrawal phenomena.

CRITERIA FOR DIAGNOSING DRUG DEPENDENCE

- A strong desire to take the substance.
- Progressive neglect of alternative sources of satisfaction.
- The development of tolerance.
- Development of withdrawal state.
- Physical and/or psychological complications.

MISUSE:

Refers to physician prescribing a drug in a medically unacceptable way.

WITHDRAWAL STATE:

A group of symptoms and signs occurring when a drug is reduced in amount or withdrawn which lasts for a limited time. There might be physical and/or psychological symptoms. The nature of the withdrawal state is related to the class of substance used.

COMMONLY ABUSED DRUGS IN INDIA:

- Alcohol
- Cannabis/ganja
- Heroin
- Opium
- Other opioids like injection pintazocaine, cough syrup.
- Prescription and OTC drugs.

Defnition:

Drug

Drug is defined as any substance that, when taken into the living organism, may modify one or more of its functions. This definition conceptualizes 'drug' in a very broad way, including not only the medications but also the other pharmacologically active substances.

There are four important patterns of drug use disorders, which may overlap with each other.

1. Acute intoxication
2. Withdrawal state
3. Dependency state and
4. Harmful use

1. Acute intoxication

According to ICD-10, acute intoxication is a transient condition following the administration of alcohol or other psychoactive substance, resulting in disturbances in level of consciousness, cognition, perception, affect or behaviour, or other psycho physiological functions and responses. This is usually associated with high blood level of the drug.

The intensity of intoxication lessens with time, and effects eventually disappear in the absence of further use of the substance. The recovery is therefore complete except where tissue damage or another complication has arisen.

2. Withdrawal state

This is characterised by a cluster of symptoms, often specific to the drug used, which develop on total or partial withdrawal of a drug, usually after repeated and/or high dose use. This, too, is a short lasting syndrome with usual duration of few hours to few days. Typically, the patients reports that withdrawal symptoms are relieved by further substance use.

The withdrawal state is further classified as

   i.   Uncomplicated
   ii.   With convulsions
   iii. With delirium

3. Dependence syndrome

According to the ICD-10, the dependence syndrome is a cluster of physiological behavioural and cognitive phenomena in which the use of a substance or a class of substances takes on a much higher priority for a given individual than other behaviours that once had greater value.

The central descriptive characteristic of the dependence syndrome is the desire (often strong, sometimes overpowering) to take psychoactive drugs (which may or may not have been medically prescribed), alcohol, or tobacco. There may be evidence that return to substance use after a period of abstinence lead to a more rapid reappearance of other features of the syndrome than occurs with nondependent individuals.

A definite diagnosis of dependence should usually be made only if at least three of the following have been experienced or exhibited at some time during the previous year:

1. A strong desire or sense of compulsion to take the substance.
2. Difficulties in controlling substance-taking behaviour in terms of its onset, termination, or levels of use.
3. A physiological withdrawal state when substance use has ceased or been reduced, as evidenced by the characteristic withdrawal syndrome for the substance; or use of the same

substance with the intention of relieving or avoiding withdrawal symptoms.
4. Evidence of tolerance, such that the increased dose of the psychoactive substance are required in order to achieve effects originally produced by lower doses.
5. Progressive neglect of alternative pleasure or interests because of psychoactive substance use, increased amount of time necessary to obtain or take the substance or to recover from its effects.
6. Persisting with substance use despite clear evidence of overtly harmful consequences

4. Harmful use
Harmful use is characterised by:
✓ Continued drug use despite awareness of harmful medical and/or social effect of the drug being used,
✓ A pattern of physically hazardous use of drug (e.g. Driving during intoxication).

The diagnosis requires that actual damage should have been caused to the mental or physical health of the user.

Psychoactive substance
The major dependence producing drugs are:
1) Alcohol
2) Opioids
3) Cannabinoids, eg. Cannabis
4) Cocaine
5) Amphetamine and other sympathomimetics
6) Hallucinogens, e.g. LSD, phencyclidine
7) Sedatives and hypnotics, EG. Barbiturates
8) Inhalants
9) Nicotine
10) Other stimulants (e.g. Caffeine)

Etiology

I. Biological factors
- Genetic vulnerability
- Co-morbid psychiatric disorder or personality disorder
- Withdrawal effects and craving
- Biochemical factors (eg. Role of dopamine and nor epinephrine in cocaine, ethanol and opoid dependence)

II. Psychological factors
➢ Curiosity; need for novelty seeking.
➢ General rebelliousness and social non conformity.
➢ Early initiation of alcohol and tobacco
➢ Poor impulse control
➢ Sensation seeking
➢ Low self-esteem.
➢ Poor stress management skills
➢ Childhood trauma or loss
➢ Relief from fatigue or boredom
➢ Escape from reality
➢ Psychological distress.

III. Social factors
✓ Peer pressure
✓ Modelling
✓ Ease of availability of alcohol and drugs. Strictness of drug law enforcement
✓ Interfamilial conflicts
✓ Poor social \ familial support
✓ Permissive social attitude
Rapid urbanization

ALCOHOL DEPENDENCE SYNDROME (ADS)

Alcoholism is a disabling addictive disorder. It is characterized by compulsive and uncontrolled consumption of alcohol despite its negative effects on the drinker's health, relationships, and social state. Heavy consumption, which involves for more than just dependence can cause untold misery to the individual, who is usually affected by other physical, psychological and social disabilities as well as elsewhere in the world. The Global Status report on alcohol and health 2014, released by the World Health Organization states that around 30% of the total population of India consumes alcohol a year

The complications of alcoholism includes depression, low self-esteem disturbed interpersonal relationships, emotional immaturity, low frustration tolerance, feeling of isolation and guilt, lack of self-confidence. Alcoholism is not only a physical problem but also a behaviour problem.

According to the American Medical Association, "Alcoholism is an illness characterized by significant impairment that is directly associated with persistent and excessive use of alcohol. Impairment may involve physiological, psychological or social dysfunction." Psychologically speaking, alcoholism has less to do with "how much" someone is drinking, and more to do with what happens when they drink. The word alcohol comes from the Arabic "Al Kohl," which means "the essence." alcohol has always been associated with rites of passages such as weddings and graduations, social occasions, sporting events and parties.

A great deal of research has been conducted concerning self-esteem and similar concept in relation to drug and alcohol use, the way the people view themselves will have an impact on how they experience their life. Their lack of self-work will affect every area of their life, especially their relationship with other people. Many of those who are dealing with low self-esteem will turn to substance abuse because it offers a temporary solution to their problem.

Alcohol use is a public health issue worldwide and a significant problem in India. Alcohol dependence is wide-spread among people of all ages and socioeconomic groups. Persons with alcohol dependence face enormous health consequences. Alcohol dependence is a major cause of mortality and is associated with psychiatric conditions, neurologic impairment, cardiovascular disease, liver disease, and malignant neoplasms. Psychiatric conditions associated with alcohol dependence include major depression, dysthymia, mania, hypomania, panic disorder, phobias, generalized anxiety disorder, personality disorders, any drug use disorder, schizophrenia, and suicide. Psychiatric comorbidity, in turn, is associated with alcohol-related symptoms of greater severity.

Excessive alcohol consumption causes brain damage, as evidenced by brain imaging, and related neurologic deficits, including impairments in working memory, cognitive processing of emotional signals, executive functions, visuospatial abilities, and gait and balance. Whereas moderate alcohol consumption is cardio protective, heavy drinking is associated with increased risks of hypertension, coronary heart disease, and ischemic stroke, possibly due to alcohol-induced sympathetic activation. Chronic excessive alcohol consumption is a strong risk factor for various types of cancer, particularly cancers of the aero-respiratory tract, but also cancers of the digestive system, liver, breast, and ovaries. Heavy drinking is associated with various forms of alcoholic liver disease, such as cirrhosis. Alcohol dependence also increases the risk of injury, possibly due to alcohol-related factors such as

13

diminished coordination and balance, increased reaction time, and impaired attention, perception, and judgment.

Alcohol also known as (ethanol) has a number of effects on health. Short-term effects of alcohol consumption include intoxication and dehydration. Long-term effects of alcohol consumption include changes in the metabolism of the liver and brain and alcoholism. Alcohol intoxication affects the brain, causing slurred speech, clumsiness, and delayed reflexes. Alcohol stimulates insulin production, which speeds up glucose metabolism and can result in low blood sugar, causing irritability and possibly death for diabetics. A 2014 Organization report found that harmful alcohol consumption caused about 3.3 million deaths annually worldwide.

The real-world impact of alcohol abuse reaches far beyond the financial costs. When a loved one has a problem with alcohol, it can affect their marriage and their extended family. There's also the larger impact on the community, schools, the workplace, the healthcare system and on society as a whole.

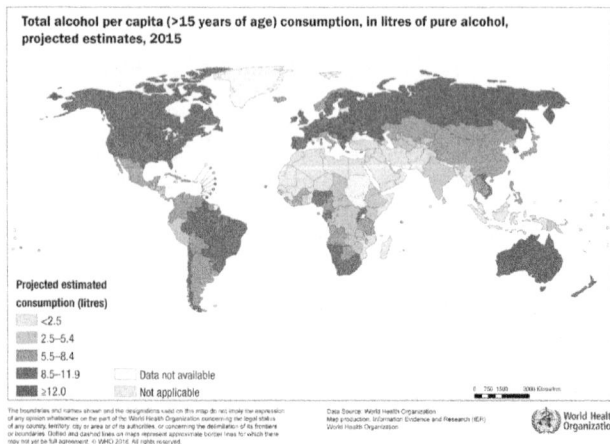

Total alcohol per capita (>15 years of age) consumption, in litres of pure alcohol, projected estimates, 2015

Projected estimated consumption (litres)
- <2.5
- 2.5–5.4
- 5.5–8.4
- 8.5–11.9
- ≥12.0
- Data not available
- Not applicable

TOTAL ALCOHOL CONSUMPTION GLOBALLY BY WHO

15 people die every day from the effects of drinking alcohol, reveals an analysis of 2013 National Crime Records Bureau data. It is estimated 2.5 million death worldwide are the result of alcohol use and 15.3 million people suffer from drug use disorder

Our brains rely on a delicate balance of chemicals and processes. Alcohol is a depressant, which means it can disrupt that balance, affecting our thoughts, feelings and actions – and sometimes our long-term mental health., when high levels of alcohol are involved, instead of pleasurable effects increasing, it's possible that a negative emotional response may occur.In India use of alcohol is higher in deprived communities contributing to 30% of use to the male population and 5% of use to female population.

Alcohol kills one Indian every 96 minutes

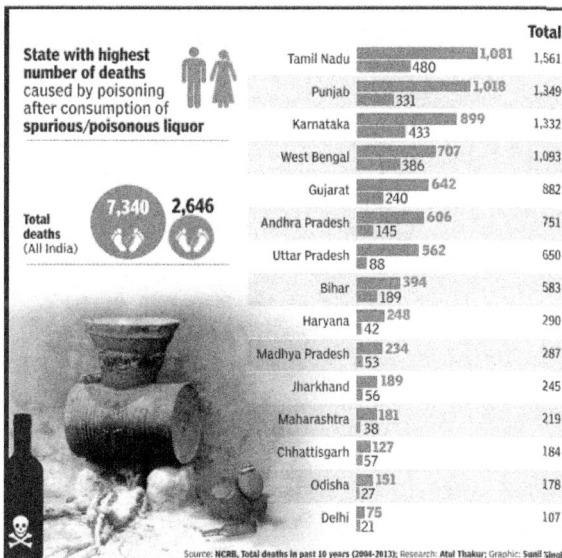

		Total
State with highest number of deaths caused by poisoning after consumption of spurious/poisonous liquor	Tamil Nadu 1,081 / 480	1,561
	Punjab 1,018 / 331	1,349
	Karnataka 899 / 433	1,332
	West Bengal 707 / 386	1,093
	Gujarat 642 / 240	882
Total deaths (All India) 7,340 / 2,646	Andhra Pradesh 606 / 145	751
	Uttar Pradesh 562 / 88	650
	Bihar 394 / 189	583
	Haryana 248 / 42	290
	Madhya Pradesh 234 / 53	287
	Jharkhand 189 / 56	245
	Maharashtra 181 / 38	219
	Chhattisgarh 127 / 57	184
	Odisha 151 / 27	178
	Delhi 75 / 21	107

Source: NCRB, Total deaths in past 10 years (2004-2013); Research: Atul Thakur; Graphic: Sunil Singh

INDIAN STATES WITH HIGHEST NUMBER OF DEATH BY CONSUMPTION OF POISONOUS LIQUOR

Indian express (2016) declared that one Indian dies every 96 minutes due to alcohol consumption.15 people die every day from the effect of drinking alcohol.

Although consuming alcohol might have become a part of the culture yet the National Crime Records Bureau (NCRB) data revealed some mind-blowing facts. In the last five years, barring 2011, there has been a continual rise in the total number of alcohol-related deaths. During the period ranging from 2009 to 2013, this figure saw a steep rise from the level of 4483 to 5518. A massive increase was alone witnessed in2011- 2012 when death figure zoomed to 5478 as against 5518 cases registered in 2013.Likewise, WHO Global status report (released in 2011) on alcohol and health stated, "The harmful use of alcohol results in approximately 2.5 million deaths each year. Almost 4 per cent of all deaths worldwide are attributed to alcohol.

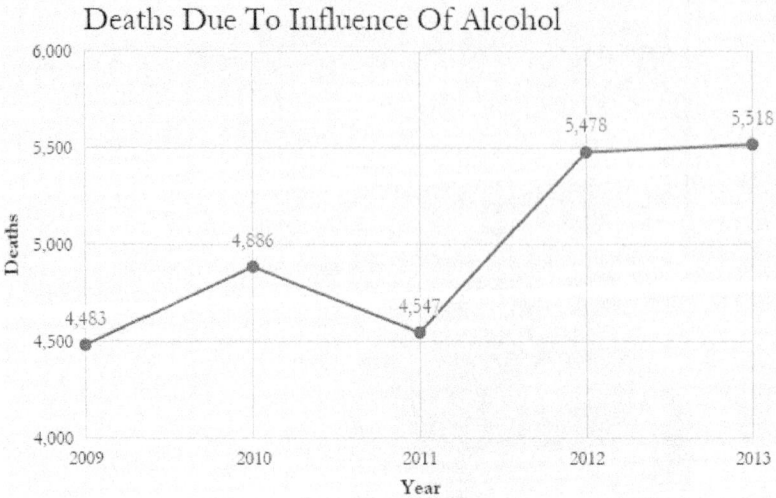

Deaths Due To Influence Of Alcohol

DEATHS DUE TO INFLUENCE OF ALCOHOL

WHO (2014) THE GLOBAL STATUS report on alcohol and health states that the amount of alcohol consumption has raised in India. The report states 38.3% of global population consume alcohol.OECD Organisation for economic co-operation and development may (2015) states 11% of Indians are moderate to heavy drinkers.3.3%death were attributed to alcohol consumption, apart from health concern, chronic concern is one of the reason for poverty in India.

Pre-poll surveys in Kerala and Tamil Nadu found wide support for prohibition, with 47% of men and women respondents in Kerala and 52% in Tamil Nadu supporting an immediate and complete ban, The Indian Express reported.

Alcoholism is a worldwide problem, not confined either to a developed or to a developing nation. Itis becoming a degenerative force in our county. Alcohol and its excessive use will affect not only the individual, but causes disorganization of family and finally lead to disintegration of the society.

Alcohol may be the most widely used drug in human history. It has been consumed for millennia worldwide for religious various cultural activities and celebration. Although judicious use of alcohol offers some benefits, recorded history as far back as the ancient Egyptians, Hindu mythology and Tamil literature like Thirukural also notes problems associated with drunkenness.The active ingredient in alcoholic drinks is ethyl alcohol. The concentration of alcohol is exposed as percentage of the volume and is variable in different alcoholic preparations.

- Beer has 8 to 11% by volume.
- Wine has 5 to 13% by volume
- Spirits 40% by volume of alcohol concentration for a standard drink.

Alcohol is observed rapidly from mouth, stomach, and small gut. Maximum blood levels reach with in an hour. Absorption is slowed down by the food and is speedened up by taking carbonated drinks.ethyl alcohol is oxidized by alcohol dehydrogenase (ADH) to acetaldehyde which in turn is oxidized by ALDH to H_2O and CO_2.Alcohol affects neuronal cell wall fluidity and permeability.

INDIA – ALCOHOLISM DURING COVID

India identified its first COVID-19 case in January 2020. To curb the spread of the pandemic, the Central Government of India declared a 21-day nationwide lockdown on 24th March 2020. The lockdown was enforced within a few hours following notification. This lockdown continued for about eight weeks and the process of unlocking was undertaken by various states in a phased manner .The sudden announcement of the lockdown led to an immediate cessation of alcohol supply in states throughout the country. This led to forced alcohol withdrawal in a substantial number of dependent alcohol users. The lack of access to acute medical care for alcohol withdrawal further compounded the situation. There were reports of suicides, accidental deaths, and increase in cases of delirium tremens or alcohol withdrawal seizures in emergency settings due to the unavailability of alcohol

The World Health Organization (WHO) estimates that alcohol consumption contributes to the world's 3 million deaths each year as well as the disability and ill health of millions of people. "Overall, alcohol abuse is a major cause of 5.1% of the world's disease burden. Alcohol is a major risk factor for premature death and disability among those aged 15 to 49, accounting for about 10 percent of all deaths in this age group. According to WHO's Global status report on alcohol and health 2018. "The highest increase is expected in the

Southeast Asian Province, with an increase of only 2.2 liters in India representing the largest population in the region," the report said. The report states that by 2018 liver disease deaths in India had reached 264,193 and accounted for 3% of all deaths. Alcohol abuse is defined as the inability to control one's drinking habits due to dependence on alcohol physically and emotionally. Drunkenness is a habit of alcohol. that often leaves your victims in a state of shock. The COVID-19 epidemic is affecting all families across the country and will likely have a lasting impact on the health and well-being of the community. Alcohol abuse has become a public health problem, and alcohol has the potential to cause the COVID-19 epidemic in many ways.

India has the highest per capita consumption of alcohol per year per 5.7 liters per person. The complex and unintended consequence of large-scale medical closures, ethical, economic, and social issues is related to alcohol consumption. After a 14-hour 'probationary period' on March 22, the Central Government announced a full closure, from March 24 to April 14, which was extended from 21 days to 3 May 2020. This was the largest closure announced since the beginning of the COVID-19 eruption, and in a country with a population of 1.3 billion, this has probably made it the largest in recorded human history. In March 2020, the World Health Organization (WHO) announced the outbreak of COVID-19 as a pandemic. During work hours during the COVID-19 epidemic, drinking alcohol can increase health risks, risky behaviors, mental health problems, and violence. Lack of access to emergency medical care when one stops drinking makes the situation worse. There have been reports of suicide, accidental death, and an increase in cases of alcoholism or emergency shocks due to a lack of alcohol. Enthusiasm led to an alcohol-disulfiram reaction . Although the emergency room claims that the reaction is caused by skin absorption, Streel and Brewer (2020) indicated in their study that the reaction may be due to inhalation of ethanol vapor rather than absorption in the skin.

EFFECT OF COVID-19 PANDEMIC AND LOCKDOWN ON PERSONS WITH ALCOHOL USE DISORDERS

PRACTICES OF DRINKING HABITS

The COVID 19 epidemic, people have drastically changed their drinking habits, switching drinking places from bars and restaurants to homes. For many people, alcohol is part of their social life, a life severely disrupted by COVID 19. After the introduction of closure, alcohol conversion is very different between young and mature adults (p <0.001). Among young people, 42% reported stable drinking behaviour compared to 76% in the adult group; 44% of young adults report drinking less compared to only 7% of mature adults. An increase in alcohol consumption has been reported in only 14% of young people and 17% of older adults. Interestingly, throughout the collection, alcohol change was most pronounced among moderate drinkers (>

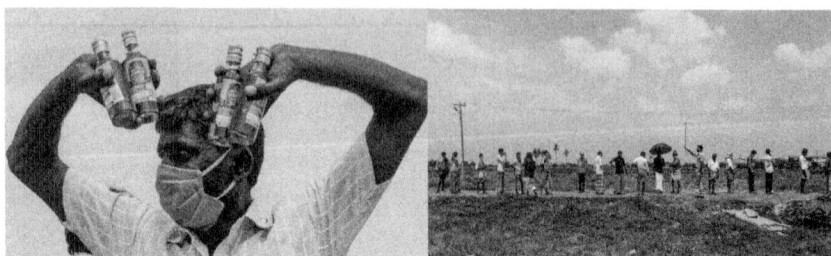

0 to <5 drinks / week) in both age groups (p <0.001). A decrease in normal status reveals female gender, lower BMI and lower age which will be associated with a decrease in the number of drinks you report /. When some Indian cities relaxed the last digestion ban to prevent the spread of the novel coronavirus, long lines appeared outside liquor stores across the country.

DOMESTIC VIOLENCE

Locks and home stay orders exacerbate some of the negative behaviours associated with harmful alcohol consumption, such as domestic violence. About 1 in 3 women will have been physically and / or sexually abused by a close partner in their lifetime, and one in three children will experience some form of violence caused by their parents or other family members The increase in violence is due to increased domestic violence, increased risk of violence, economic burden, and limited access to survivors to support services available prior to housing closure. The COVID-19 response system limited the spread of the virus, however, weakening women's ability to respond to their violent abusers. During the violence, there was an increase in the number of emergency calls to help report domestic violence.

HEALTH-RELATED ISSUES

Alcohol withdrawal syndrome (AWS) usually occurs after stopping strong or persistent strong or indirect drinking. Although the most common symptoms of AWS include tremors, sweating, etc., 15% of those with AWS experience severe symptoms such as epilepsy and delirium tremens (DT). Death rates for those with severe alcohol withdrawal (20%) these can be significantly reduced to less than 1% with early detection and appropriate treatment for people who die accidentally as a result of taking alcohol-based antibiotics, or self-inflicted injuries as a result of the trauma resulting from this condition. The announced closure to prevent the spread of Covid 19 in India has created unforeseen problems, including severe withdrawal symptoms and the need for self-regulation. The state of Kerala in India witnessed the suicide of six victims, prompting the state government to order state doctors to administer alcohol to drug addicts. The local medical association went to court against this. These events raise exciting moral issues.

ALCOHOL DISEASES

Sudden closure and ban on alcohol in many countries has seen a sudden increase in complex alcohol withdrawal. There have also been reports of alcohol withdrawal leading to suicidal incidents during the COVID-19 violence in India, creating potential problems for non-communication. There have been cases in which doctors have ordered alcohol consumption to be controlled, which in turn has led to behavioural problems. Of particular concern, in the absence of legal alcohol, have been the use of methanol or household products that lead to youthful methanol, Serious complications, including blindness, putamen necrosis, bleeding of subcortical white matter and even death have been reported. In the wake of the coronavirus 2019 violence (COVID-19), many regions around the world have recommended orders for residency, closure of public places, and physical isolation to reduce community spread. These measures have contributed to isolation and anxiety, with recent studies showing an increase in alcohol consumption that followed. Although alcohol consumption can lead to temporary relief of stress, alcohol abuse is a leading cause of death worldwide, contributing to about 3 million deaths a year.

CHANGES IN ALCOHOL CONSUMPTION

During this epidemic, there has been an increase in addiction-related behaviours. Research suggests an increase in alcohol, marijuana and tobacco, screening time, behavioural addiction, high salt intake, and high-calorie foods. As expected, there has been an increase in health-related behaviours such as physical inactivity, sedentary lifestyle,

EFFECTS OF CO-MORBID MEDICAL CROSS

Sick diseases increase the risk of death in patients with COVID-19. In patients with alcohol-related liver disease, excessive alcohol consumption may increase new liver failure. During treatment, patients with alcohol-induced hepatitis B may develop an increased risk of COVID-19 infection. High mortality has been observed in patients with alcohol-related liver disease and COVID-19. In a study in India, patients with cirrhosis of the liver infected with COVID-19 had serious side effects, with the worst effects among those presenting with chronic liver failure In this study, one third of the patients had alcohol. In addition, alcohol-induced liver disease was found to be an independent risk of death following the dietary habits of COVID-19 which also changed during COVID-19 and was associated with changes in alcohol consumption A Lithuanian study found that alcohol consumption was associated with an increase. weight gain In a study in Japan, people who drank alcohol and who lived a sedentary lifestyle after working on a telephone, had a high risk of developing diabetes.

SUICIDE AND CLOSURE

More than 8,000 suicide bombers in India during the closure of COVID-2020. India Introduces "Total Lockdown" After Spike in Cases ', 2020), later extended to 3 May (' PM Narendra Modi Says India Will Extend Coronavirus Closure Until 3 May ', 2020) However, India saw another problem due to the closure. Most of the liquor stores are currently closed following a government proclamation that led to alcoholism (AWS) .So, from 5 May 2020, at least 23 people committed suicide along with a few others who attempted suicide as a result of alcohol shortcomings and AWS. All these people came from the southern states of India, namely, Kerala, Tamil Nadu, Telangana, and Karnataka. The number of patients with AWS visiting various mental health hospitals for consultation has increased at least four times during the closure of COVID-19 compared to normal days throughout India.

ALCOHOL AND DANGER OF RECEIVING COVID-19

'Alcohol consumption' among alcohol users increases COVID-19 tendency and alcohol use during COVID-19 infection has been described as a 'dangerous cocktail' In a Spanish-based observational study, among 2078 COVID-19 patients tested throughout. 3 months, the prevalence of SUDs was 1.3%, mainly for men (85%). At 1.3%, alcohol is the most widely consumed substance in two-thirds. It has been suggested that chronic alcohol use increases the risk of COVID-19 by reducing infection, increasing the inflammatory response, and related liver disease. Recent reviews suggest an increased risk of infection in people with all SUDs. chronic alcohol use as a potential risk factor for SARS-CoV-2 infection. Drinking Alcohol Increases Risk Of COVID-19 .

ALCOHOL DISABLES THE SELF-PROGRAM

Drinking alcohol can change the amount, survival, and function of many immune cells. Although these changes alone may not be enough to have a negative impact on a person's health, if a person is exposed to a second "hit", such as a virus, his or her immune system may not respond properly, increasing the risk of infection. The specific effects of alcohol on the immune system depend largely on how often and how much a person drinks . Alcohol abuse makes the body more susceptible to infections and can be worse than prognosis. Alcohol in the body during exposure to the pathogen often disrupts the body's immediate response to the pathogen, making it easier for the infection to progress. For a long time, excessive use of alcohol interferes with the function of the immune system in the lungs, causing the body's immune system to malfunction. Excessive alcohol consumption also damages the cells around the lungs and the damage may remain undiagnosed until disease develops in the lungs.

EASY IN DESTROYED FARMING

About one third of all patients with ulcers such as burns, broken bones, and brain damage and other tissues have high blood pressure levels above the legal limit at the time of injury. Alcohol abuse not only increases the risk of such injuries, but may adversely affect the outcomes of these patients. These effects appear to be considered primarily in changes in immune function, making patients at greater risk for subsequent immune challenges, such as surgery or infection. As a result, these patients are more likely to die during recovery. Alcohol abuse is especially dangerous for people with burn injuries. About 50 percent of burnout patients have significant levels of alcohol in their blood when hospitalized. These patients have more problems, require longer hospital stays, and have a higher rate of death compared to non-drunk patients at the time of injury. Patients with burn injuries are at risk of developing lung diseases. Alcohol intoxication during injury increases the risk of such diseases by suppressing the immune system. Similarly, both burns and alcohol damage disrupt the intestinal tract, allowing germs to enter the bloodstream and increase risk.

POLICIES AND LAWS

Existing alcohol control policies and programs in India have not been fully effective in controlling the burden of alcohol use and its related effects. There is a need for a comprehensive, evidence-based and co-ordinated national alcohol control policy to effectively guide and support Indian countries in alcohol control and reduce associated burden. The effective implementation of such policies is crucial to its success. Alcohol is a topic on the State list under Schedule Seventh of the Constitution of India. Therefore, the rules governing alcohol vary from state to state. There have been major changes in the global liquor policy regarding the epidemic. Although many countries ban alcohol, some have declared alcohol to be 'essential'. Both policy positions have led to public health concerns and legal issues with increasing alcohol withdrawal, use of pesticides, methanol poisoning due to illicit alcohol use, and alcohol misuse for medical purposes. in restricted countries. In lands where alcohol consumption was considered relatively high, this resulted in an increase in home-based alcoholic beverages. A representative of the changes in alcohol trends during the closure of Google courses. Google's Google analysis in India compares premature closures, 1.0 locks and 2.0 locks. Compared to pre-closure closures, there was a significant increase in online searches for distilled spirits (not beer), access to alcohol, and alcohol withdrawal during the 1.0 closure (21 day). However, during the second phase of lockdown

2.0, compared to pre-lockdown closures, there was an increase in demand for benzodiazepines related words. These findings indicate that the initial search was focused on alcohol intake and later on access to extended alcohol-related withdrawal treatment. A similar Google trend analysis suggests an increase in search terms after alcohol closures related to alcohol withdrawal and purchase methods, reflecting changes in trends.

EFFECTS OF ADDICTIONAL MEDICINE SERVICES

In India, during the initial closure period, less than 20% of registered drunk patients were able to receive treatment. It was considered difficult to obtain withdrawal control assistance and access to recurrent anti-retroviral drugs (such as Disulfiram. Admission to rehabilitation centres was severely affected, as suggested by experience from India, where many were closed during closure and some used had a COVID-19 outbreak, due to overuse. Strict safety measures. During the COVID-19 epidemic, many medical and disaster risk reduction organizations have had to reduce their hours and services for people with substance abuse, putting these people at increased risk of death. From the Abuse Mental Health Services Administration, the US Drug Enforcement Administration, and the US Department of Health and Human Services have approved the use of audio- telehealth integration only the introduction of buprenorphine without the need for personal testing or video interface. This has empowered new strategies to try and meet the needs of those most at risk during the current epidemic.

OPPORTUNITY FOR TREATMENT

Several doctors have described shutting down the door as an "treatment option" for alcoholics. According to a newspaper report, a document produced by the National Drug Dependence Treatment Centre, the All India Institute of Medical Sciences

(AIIMS), called the closure situation a blessing for some people who could use the opportunity to stop drinking altogether changes in health care service delivery -19 created both challenges and opportunities for all patients with substance abuse disorders including virtual or telemedicine visits, medication access problems and ensuring access to naloxone where supplies cannot be provided. Unique challenges in pregnant and postpartum patients with substance abuse include further evidence of reduced access to medication for opioid use problems and changes in birth control that separate birth attendants from supportive caregivers. The possibilities for all patients with substance abuse problems include visual forums that present good opportunities for treatment. They work well on time, remove transport barriers, and can reduce barriers.

SCREENING TEST FOR ALCOHOLISM

C Have you ever felt you ought to cut down on your drinking?

A Have people annoyed you by criticizing your drinking?

G Have you ever felt bad or guilty about your drinking?

E Have you ever had a drink first thing in the morning to steady your nerves or get rid of a hangover (eye opener)?

Positive replies to any two of these questions, it is understood that the person is abusing alcohol and need further proper drinking history to confirm alcoholism.

THE PROCESS OF DEVELOPMENT OF ALCOHOLISM:

Experimental	To begin with, persons start drinking alcohol due to peer pressure and curiosity
Recreational	Gradually, whenever they meet in festivals, functions like marriages, hostel day or college day, parties, conferences, they drink occasionally.
Relaxational	Further, whenever they want relaxation, on holidays and week ends, they start enjoying their drink and continue to do so. Hence the frequency gradually increases.
Compulsive	Some people who started drinking occasionally, start drinking almost daily or drinking heavily for a period of time for pleasure or to avoid the discomfort of withdrawal symptoms.

ETIOLOGY OF ADS:

1)   Biological Factors:
Genetic factors play an important role. First-degree relatives of alcoholics have double the risk of the disorder. The inheritance seems to be polygenic.

2)   Biochemical:
•   Release of dopamine in the mesolimbic system brings euphoria and inhibition of glutaminergic transmission mediates amnesic effects.
•   Alcohol increases GABA – transmission, which is responsible for its anxiolytics action.

3) Psychological Factors:
Alcohol abuse is quite common in antisocial and borderline personality
disorders. Persons with chronic pain, insomnia, depression, and anxiety disorders often seek relief through drug use. Behavioral scientists view drug abuse has a maladaptive learned behavior.

4) Social Factors:
Increased societal tolerance, decreased restrictions, and easy availability of alcohol are associated with high prevalence states.

5) The Pharmacological
Properties of the drug itself may contribute to abuse. Availability, accessibility, and affordability are other important reasons.

SCREENING OF ALCOHOLISM

Detection of alcoholism can be made by asking alcohol screening questions.

Questions that people who work in the field of alcohol addiction often ask:

- Do you drink because you have problems or to relax?
- Do you prefer to drink alone, rather than with other people?
- Is your work or education suffering as a result of your drinking?
- Have you ever tried to stop drinking, or to drink less, and found that you can't?
- Do you drink in the morning, before school or work?
- Do you ever have loss of memory due to your drinking?
- Do you lie about how much or how often you drink?
- Do other people comment on your drinking and think it's a problem?

If you answer 'yes' to any of these questions, it's important that you talk to someone about your drinking. Facing up to the fact that you might have a problem takes courage. Deciding to get some help is a really brave move, but it can be one of the best things ever do.There is no safe level of drug use. Use of any drug always carries some risk. It's important to be careful when taking any type of drug.

Alcohol affects everyone differently, based on:

- Size, weight and health
- Whether the person is used to taking it
- Whether other drugs are taken around the same time
- The amount drunk
- The strength of the drink

The following day after drinking alcohol,   the client may have a hangover. Its effects include:

- Headache
- Diarrhoea And Nausea
- Tiredness And Trembling
- Increased Heart Rate And Blood Pressure
- Dry Mouth
- Trouble Concentrating
- Anxiety
- Poor Or Decreased sleep.

LONG-TERM EFFECTS

- Regular Use Of Alcohol May Eventually Cause:
- Depression
- Poor Memory And Brain Damage

- Difficulty Getting An Erection
- Difficulty Having Children
- Liver Disease
- Cancer
- High Blood Pressure And Heart Disease
- Needing To Drink More To Get The Same Effect
- Physical dependence on alcohol.

Alcohol and mental health

Research shows a relationship between people who are dependent on alcohol and increased mental health issues. People with mental health issues may drink more alcohol to self-medicate. This can lead to longer-term anxiety and depression.

Tolerance and dependence

People who regularly use alcohol can become dependent on the drug. They may feel they need alcohol to go about their normal activities like working, studying and socialising, or just to get through the day.They may also develop a tolerance to it, which means they need to drink larger amounts of alcohol to get the same effect. People who develop a tolerance and dependence on alcohol experience more alcohol-related harms.

Mixing alcohol with other drugs

- The effects of drinking and taking other drugs − including over-the-counter or prescribed medications − can be unpredictable and dangerous, and could cause:
- Alcohol + cannabis: nausea, vomiting, panic, anxiety and paranoia.

- Alcohol + energy drinks (with caffeine), ice, speed or ecstasy: more risky behaviour, body under great stress, overdose more likely.
- Alcohol + GHB or benzodiazepines: decreased heart rate, overdose more likely.

SIGNS OF ALCOHOL ABUSE

Sometimes it can be hard to notice when a regular couple of drinks has turned into too many, too often. The fact that thinking about whether to have a problem is a good start. There are some signs of alcohol dependence that can look out for.

Mental and social signs include:

Worrying about when to have next drink, or wanting to, when to wake up in the morning consuming alcohol regularly on own, or trying to hide drinking from those around worsening relationships with friends or family, always staying out late and encouraging friends to keep drinking when they've said they want to go home.

Physical signs include:

- Sweating
- Feeling Nauseous
- Unable To Get To Sleep Without Drinking Alcohol
- Need to drink more and more alcohol to get drunk.

PHYSICAL COMPLICATIONS OF ALCOHOL ABUSE:

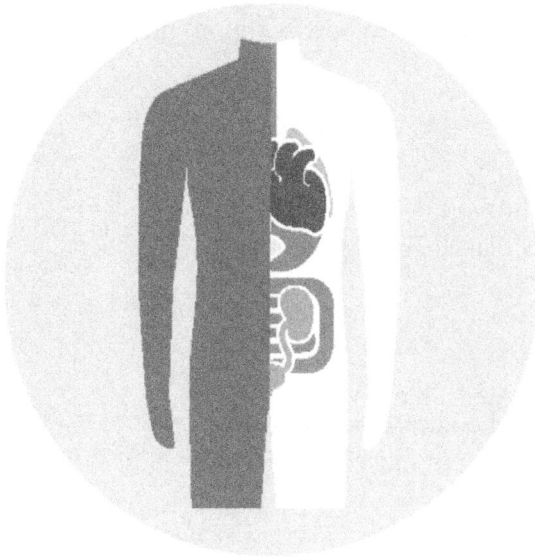

GASTROINTESTINAL

- Dyspepsia
- Vomiting
- Acute or chronic gastritis
- Peptic ulcer
- Cancer

LIVER

- Fatty degeneration of the liver
- Alcoholic hepatitis
- Cirrhosis
- Carcinoma of liver

PANCREAS

- Acute and chronic Pancreatitis

CARDIOVASCULAR

- Alcoholic Cardiomyopathy
- High risk for myocardial infarction

BLOOD

- Folic acid deficiency anaemia
- Decreased WBC production.

MUSCLE

- Peripheral muscle weakness
- Wasting of muscles

SKIN

- Spider angiomas
- Acne

NUTRITION

- Protein malnutrition
- Vitamin deficiency disorder like pellagra and beriberi

JOINTS

- Gout due to increase in uric acid level

REPRODUCTIVE SYSTEM

- Sexual dysfunction in males
- Failure of ovulation in females

PREGNANCY

- Fetal alcohol syndrome – fetal abnormalities like mental retardation and growth deficiency.

NERVOUS SYSTEM

- Alcoholic peripheral neuropathy
- Wernicke's- Korsakoff syndrome

PSYCHIATRIC COMPLICATIONS OF ALCOHOL ABUSE:

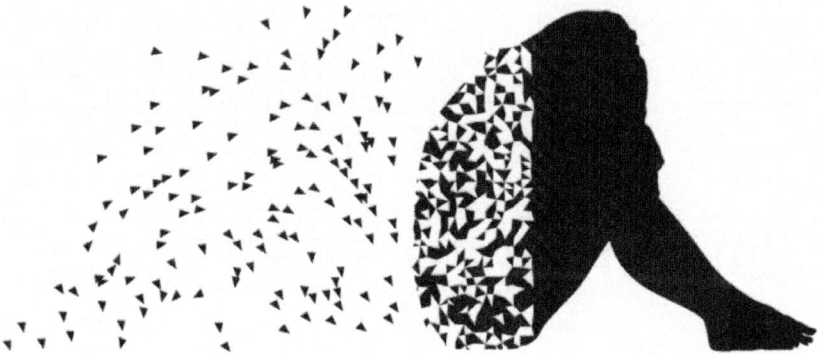

Pathological intoxication maladaptive behavioural effects, such as fighting, impaired judgement, physiological signs such as slurred speech, inco ordination, unsteady gait, and psychological changes such as mood changes, irritability and impaired attention.

Withdrawal phenomenon The general withdrawal symptoms are:

- Tremor
- Nausea And Vomiting
- Malaise
- Tachycardia
- Elevated B.P
- Irritability,
- Anorexia
- Insomnia
- Fits.

Delirium tremens (DT) is a complicated withdrawal state. An acute organic mental disorder and this should be treated as a psychiatric emergency. DT is a short-lived, but occasionally life-threatening, toxic, confusional state with accompanying somatic disturbance. Prodromal symptoms are insomnia, tremulousness and fear, and occasionally convulsions. The classical features are:

a. Altered consciousness and confusion
b. Auditory and visual Hallucination and illusions
c. Marked tremor and fever
d. Delusion, agitation, increased ANS activities.

Treatment:

Hospitalization, IV fluids, inj.thiamine and other B-complex and multi vitamins, benzodiazepines to reduce agitation and restlessness and to prevent withdrawal fits (Rum fits).

Alcoholic psychosis

Person drinking alcohol for a long time and in large quantities are prone to develop a psychotic disorder which resembles paranoid schizophrenia with clinical features like behavioural problems, thought disturbance, delusions, hallucinations and impairment of primary mental functions.

Delusional disorder

Delusional disorder (Morbid jealosy or Othello syndrome)A paranoid disorder with predominal delusion of infedility of spouse (Suspecting wife's character)

Alcoholism and depression

Alcoholics are more prone to develop depression. To get relief from depression some people drink, which will further aggravate the depression. Attempted suicide and suicide are more common in alcoholics.

Alcoholism and criminality

Alcohol reduces inhibition and increase hostile behaviour. Hence alcoholics are more prone to violence and antisocial behaviour.

Alcoholism and Sex

Alcohol increases the sexual desire but takes away the performance. Alcoholic males suffer from sexual dysfunction.

Alcohol amnestic disorder

Impairment in short and long-term memory with disorientation and confabulation.

Alcoholic dementia

A chronic organic mental disorder due to long-term alcohol drinking. Irreversible impairment in memory, orientation, impulse control, ability to solve problems etc. may be there.

SOCIAL COMPLICATIONS OF ALCOHOLISM:

Work problems

Decreased work performance, hence decreased productivity Absenteeism. As a result, the economy of the nation suffers.

Family problems

Alcoholism is a disease which not only affects the individual but his whole family. Loss of job, loss of income will make the family condition miserable. There will be a role model reversal, i.e. the bread-winner becomes an alcoholic and the wife takes the role of earning. Marital disharmony is a common complication.Drunken drivingWill lead to accidents. Street quarrels causing nuisance to public.

SELF ESTEEM IN ALCOHOLISM

Alcohol and self-esteem mutually impact one another. Alcohol use can temporarily raise or lower self-esteem, but it typically creates lower self-esteem in the long-term. Low or high self-esteem can be a contributing factor to alcohol abuse and dependence, but an appropriate level of self-esteem is a powerful tool in the battle against alcoholism.Alcohol and self-esteem has a mutually destructive relationship. As a chemical depressant, alcohol can negatively impact one's mental state, especially if they suffer from an external disorder or factors that affect their self-esteem

Alcoholism, or the dependence on and compulsive consumption of alcohol, is a serious disease that can have serious consequences. but oftentimes it can also lead to legal problems and criminal charges, such as driving under the influence. Furthermore, it can cause serious physical and mental health issues.

Alcoholism and Low Self-Esteem

Self-esteem is defined as the way we view ourselves. Individuals with high self-esteem tend to view themselves in a positive light and have high confidence levels. In contrast, individuals with low self-esteem tend to have negative images of themselves and lack the ability to believe in their own self-worth and abilities.

Low self-esteem is often seen in individuals who have problems with alcohol. Although self-esteem tends to increase in the beginning stages of alcoholism, it eventually tends to decrease as alcoholics become more and more isolated and lose connections with people who used to be important in their lives. This decrease in self-esteem can lead alcoholics to accept that they will never escape addiction, thereby preventing them from seeking help. Some symptoms of low self-esteem include the following:

- Believing that others view in a negative light
- Feeling unable to succeed at anything
- Having negative thoughts about oneself
- Thinking that others are out to get
- Entering into or staying in bad relationships

Low self-esteem has been linked to the onset of drug use, and research has also shown a connection between low self-esteem and behavioral addictions including internet addiction, eating problems, and compulsive buying. While alcohol, drugs, or compulsive behaviors can initially mask insecurities and even make people feel more confident, these feelings are short-lived. Over time, grappling with the effect of addiction can harm a person's self-esteem and make recovery more difficult. Whether you're contemplating doing something about your addiction, or you're already on the road to recovery, these five exercises can help rebuild your self-esteem and improve your well-being and outlook on life.

Signs of alcoholism
Some of the signs of alcoholism include the following:

- Inability to stay in control of drinking alcohol
- Inability to refrain from drinking alcohol
- Suffering from shaking, sweating, and mood swings when you stop drinking alcohol
- Alcohol use interferes with the ability to maintain a job or relationship
- Withdrawal from hobbies and responsibilities so you can drink
- Drinking alcohol secretly
- Having the urge to drink alcohol as soon as you wake up
- Not remembering what happened while on a drinking binge

The Relationship between Alcohol and Self-Esteem

Alcoholism Triggered by Unhealthy Self-Esteem
Alcohol abuse goes hand-in-hand with a harmful self-esteem. Self-esteem that is too low or high can be a trigger for someone to start drinking. Though they are for opposite reasons, both lead to a potential for dependency.

Filling the Void of Low Self-Esteem with Alcohol
People who battle low self-esteem hold themselves with little regard. They don't believe that their thoughts or opinions hold as much value as others' and that they won't have the same level of success as those close to them. Low self-esteem can be an issue in its own right, or it can be the result of a number of different personality disorders, such as Borderline Personality Disorder.

Reinforcing Fragile High Self-Esteem with Alcohol

People with fragile high self-esteem can often be identified by them hinging their self-worth on their performance in regular tasks. Failure can be a trigger for them to start using or become aggressive at others, trying to tear them down to feel better about Treatment for Alcohol and Self-Esteem Issues

Promoting Self Esteem In Alcoholism

Write Your Own Affirmation

An affirmation is a simple, positive statement to say to oneself. While affirmations may not seem genuine at first, reciting them eventually does change the way one feel about oneself. Write an affirmation that reflects how one want to feel about oneself, One study found that in individuals with low self-esteem, self-affirmations helped improve their attitudes toward health risk advice. This might be particularly helpful for people who are working to recover from a substance or alcohol use disorder. Affirmations may help people feel more receptive and motivated to participate in treatment and recovery.

Forgive one for Past Mistakes

People who have struggled with an addiction are often plagued by self-blame, which worsens low self-esteem. Addiction can really affect judgment and impulse control, . never let past wrongs define your present. Research also supports the importance of self-forgiveness. Studies suggest that people who forgive themselves for past mistakes experience less anxiety and depression.4

Accept Compliments

Research has shown that people who have low self-esteem have a difficult time accepting and benefiting from compliments from other people. This is challenging not only for a person's self-esteem but also makes it harder for people who care about that individual to express their positive feelings for that person. People with low self-esteem often miss opportunities to build their self-esteem simply by acknowledging the kind words of others. Some things you can do instead the next time someone gives you a compliment include:

- Resist the urge to dismiss it.
- Assume that they are sincere.
- Say thank you and enjoy the compliment.
- Note how the compliment reflects your strengths.

Do Something Kind Every Day

Research also suggests that engaging in prosocial behavior, or actions designed to benefit others, can also play a role in improving self-esteem. One study found that prosocial behavior was actually a predictor for self-esteem, especially in women. Women who reported engaging in more prosocial actions also had higher levels of self-reported self-esteem. One way of increasing the appreciation that others express t is to do kind things for them.

Start Making Changes

Self-determination can also play a role in improving self-esteem. Self-determined behaviors are those that people perform of their own volition as a result of conscious, intentional, self-motivated choices.Self-determination is also an important part of recovery from substance and alcohol use.. Making self-determined steps in the right direction—even small ones—can play a role in boosting your self-esteem. Everyone has things they would like to change in their own lives, or in the lives of those around them, but for people with addictions, change happens in stages.If a major change seems like too much, break it down into smaller acts, and choose to do one a day or one a week, whichever you feel you'll follow through on. With each small change, inwardly celebrate your success in moving toward your goal.

Counselling in alcoholism

Counselling is a talking therapy that allows people to discuss their problems with trained professionals in a peaceful and safe ambiance, it is the process about talking issues in detail either intending to overcome the same or to explore thoughts comprehensively. Counselors and clients both be aware that the counseling process requires patience In addition, the counseling process is collaborative. The counselor does not fix the client; the work requires interaction and commitment from both parties

DEFINITION

Counselling

- The process that occurs when a client and counsellor set aside time to explore difficulties which may include the stressful or emotional feelings of the client.

- The act of helping the client to see things more clearly, possibly from a different viewpoint. This can enable the client to focus on feelings, experiences or behavior, with a goal of facilitating positive change.

METHODS OF COUNSELLING

In-Person: Face-to-face

Counselling sessions take place in the counselor's chamber where both of them meet in person after scheduling an appointment to discuss problems. It is one of the most popular counselling formats.

Group Counselling:

Professionals provide group counselling sessions where to address the issues. Joining such a group will help to find people with similar problems and will be able to develop a strong network of support as well.

Telephonic Sessions: A great alternative to in-person counselling sessions are telephonic rounds that can be scheduled from the comfort of home. Telephonic counselling rounds are best for busy individuals who might find it difficult to get into the chambers. Online Counselling, also known as e-therapy, e-counseling, teletherapy, or cyber-counseling, involves providing mental health services and support over the internet. Services can be offered through email, text messaging, video conferencing, online chat, messaging, or internet phone.

COUNSELLING PROCESS

The counselling process involves a step-by-step approach and the counselor conducts it in a way to make sure that the client is comfortable with the process. There are five crucial stages of a counselling process.

Building a Warm Relationship

Building a lasting relationship with clients starts at the very beginning. there are steps need to take from the relationship for success like to know them, establish preferred communication channels, foster open communication, treat client like a person, ask for feedback. Analysis In this stage, the professional encourages to speak in detail about problems to grab the roots of the problem. Counselors observes every minute detail from speaking to reactions to certain questions that might come from end. Once he assesses the problem, the goal is fixed.

Setting the Goal

After a thorough evaluation of problems, now comes the significant section of goal setting. Considering the issues, the counselor sets a goal. That can be either overcoming the problem or reconciling with it.

Plan of Action

The counselor plans an action for to practice to see the results. Suppose someone has public speaking fear, The expert might ask him to practice speaking in front of the mirror. He assesses improvement. If things seem normal, He plan for final stage If not, he might design something different. Overcoming the Problem After following the plan of action, the consequent results are taken into consideration. If things seem to go in the right direction and the client start feeling relaxed, the goal is achieved.

COUNSELLING SKILLS

Being a professional counselor requires some core skills to be able to handle client queries and drive the best results for them. The vital skills that a professional counselor must have are as follows:

• **Effective Listening**: A counselor must be a patient listener who not only listens to the clients queries but can handle them intricately. Without hearing the issues minutely, it is impossible to get ahead with the next counselling steps.

• **A Good Communicator**: A counselor is someone who listens to his clients, analyses the problems, and develops a plan of action to achieve a target.

• **Analysis**: A successful counselor is someone who is not only a good listener but a good analyzer too, who uses his skills and expertise to reach the root of the problem and analyze it.

TYPES OF COUNSELLING

The counselling types are numerous and here we will be discussing a few of them.

Mental Health Counselling

A mental health counselor is responsible for providing the people with support through any emotional distress like fear of something, anxiety, depression, or frustration.

Career Counselling

A career counselling means providing aspirants with career guidance and showing them the right path towards a bright career according to their areas of interest and skills. The career counselling curriculum is designed to guide people in selecting, changing, or leaving a career and can be availed at any stage of life.

Rehabilitation Counselling

The rehabilitation counselling process helps people with disabilities fulfill their goals and lead an independent life with complete participation in the community. This is a systematic method to help people with emotional, physical, cognitive, and mental disabilities accomplish their life goals and live cherishable life.

Relationship Counselling

It is also known as couples therapy; people seek such counselling when something serious affects their love life. People choose to go for relationship counselling for various reasons including the desire to have a stronger relationship with the partner or spouse, issues emerging from disagreement, unhealthy abuses, something hectic that affected their lives, etc

THE STAGES OF THE COUNSELING PROCESS

The counseling process is a planned and structured dialogue between client and counselor. The counselor is a trained and qualified professional who helps the client identify the source of their concerns or difficulties; then, together, they find counseling approaches to help deal with the problems faced.

Stage one: (Initial disclosure) Relationship building The counseling process begins with relationship building. This stage focuses on the counselor engaging with the client to explore the issues that directly affect them.The vital first interview can set the scene for what is to come, with the client reading the counselor's verbal and nonverbal signals to draw inferences about the counselor and the process. The counselor focuses on using good listening skills and building a positive relationship.

Stage two: (In-depth exploration) Problem assessment The counselor carefully listens and draws out information regarding the client's situation and the reason they have engaged in counseling. Information crucial to subsequent stages of counseling includes identifying triggers, timing, environmental factors, stress levels, and other contributing factors.

Stage three: (Commitment to action) Goal setting Effective counseling relies on setting appropriate and realistic goals, building on the previous stages. The goals must be identified and developed collaboratively, with the client committing to a set of steps leading to a particular outcome.

Stage four: Counseling intervention This stage varies depending on the counselor and the theories they are familiar with, as well as the situation the client faces.

Stage five: Evaluation, termination, or referral Termination may not seem like a stage, but the art of ending the counseling is critical. Drawing counseling to a close must be planned well in advance to ensure a positive conclusion is reached while avoiding anger, sadness, or anxiety.

MANAGEMENT OF ALCOHOLISM

Advice for people who have had a stroke

Alcohol can increase the risk of having another one. It can increase the impact of changes to speech, thinking, vision and balance caused by stroke. Alcohol can interfere with some medicines and can be harmful.

Change drinking

While drinking, keep count of how many standard drinks to have. Make a note in a book or on phone if need to.

In social situations:

- Drink slowly and make every second drink a non-alcoholic drink. Choose sparkling water rather than a sugary drink.
- Drink low-alcohol drinks such as light beer or one of the many non-alcoholic beer, wine and spirits now available.
- Say "I'm not drinking" or "I've had one already thanks". You don't need to explain or justify your decision not to drink alcohol.

Get help

Talk with your doctor about treatment and counselling services.Counselling Online is a free and confidential service that provides support to people affected by alcohol or drug use. Health professionals provide information, advice, support and referral. Practical and confidential advice will help you manage your health better and live well.

An Unhealthy Relationship with Alcohol

On the flip side, there are a couple of identifiers which may signify that a person has an unhealthy relationship with alcohol. Using alcohol to cope with uncomfortable situations,life events, feelings or emotions

- Hiding alcohol use
- Drinking alone
- Alcohol becomes a priority over your responsibilities (e.g. work, school, etc.)
- Experiencing guilt over drinking

- Strained relationships due to behaviour under the influence of alcohol
- Participating in risky behaviour as a result of drinking (e.g. drink driving, unprotected sex)
- Dependence and withdrawal symptoms (e.g. needing more alcohol to experience the same effects)
- Losing control of drinking – not being able to stop even if you want to
- Drinking and the after effects (e.g. recovering from a hangover) start to take over life.

- People who have taken over-the-counter or prescription medication.
- People suffering from liver, heart or pancreatic diseases.

I. Assessment of the patient.
- Family and work environment, other psychosocial stressors.
- Detailed history of drinking pattern.
- Comorbid physical and psychological disorders.

II. Physical method of treatment.

DETOXIFICATION

Detoxification is the process by which an alcohol dependent person recovers from the intoxicating effects of alcohol in a supervised way. It includes:

- Administration of anti-anxiety drugs like chlordiazepoxide or lorazepram to reduce withdrawal symptoms and to control insomnia agitation and tremors.
- Vitamin supplements especially inj.thiamine in large quantity.
- Rehydration – to correct any electrolyte imbalance.

- Glucose – to correct any hypoglycaemia
- Antibiotics – to treat any infection
- Pharmacological treatments for the maintenance of abstinence after detoxification:

a) Disulfiram(250mg tablets)– an aversive stimulus, including nausea in the patient if alcohol is consumed; efficacy limited by problems with compliance (patients who wish to start drinking again tend to stop the Disulfiram to avoid the nausea).

b) Acamprosate(Acamptas 333mg tablets) - works on the GABA / glutamate system, the maintenance of abstinence. Good choice for patient's with mild to moderate hepatic impairment.

c) Naltrexone (50mg tablets) – opiate receptors antagonize for the maintenance of abstinence.

NB:Both Acamprosate and Naltrexone are associated with less side affects, do not interact with alcohol and non-addictive and in combinationthey are useful agents to enhance relapse prevention.

III. PSYCHOLOGICAL THERAPIES
- Counseling
- Individual and group psychotherapy.
- Marital and family therapy.
- Behaviour modification.
- Relapse prevention therapy.

IV. REHABILITATION – long term management with focused occupation therapy.

V. ALCOHOLIC ANONYMOUS (AA)

A self group of ex-addicts, who confront, instruct and support fellow -drinkers in their efforts to stay sober one day at a time, through fellow ship and acceptance. The Australian guidelines are based on a 'standard drink'. Not many people know how to measure a standard drink. The size of a standard drink depends on drinking:

- Spirits: 30 ml of spirits with 40% alcohol by volume is 1 standard drink.
- Beer: A 285 ml glass of full-strength beer is 1.1 standard drinks. A 285 ml glass of low-strength beer is 0.6 standard drinks. 285 ml is a small glass of beer.
- Wine: 100 ml of wine or champagne is about 1 standard drink. The average glass in restaurants and pubs is 150 ml.

The label states how many standard drinks are in the bottle.

What is a standard drink?

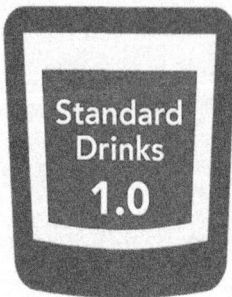

What does a standard drink look like?

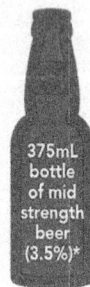

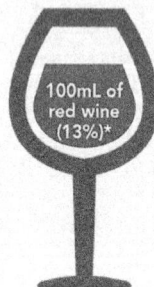

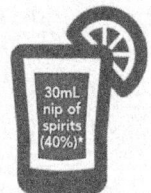

Standard Drinks 1.0 =

375mL bottle of mid strength beer (3.5%)*

100mL of red wine (13%)*

30mL nip of spirits (40%)*

* This information is a guide only and has been sourced from the Australian Government Department of Health at alcohol.gov.au

OPIOID USE DISORDERS

Dried exudates obtained from unripe seed capsules of papaversomniferum has been used and abused for centuries. The most important dependence producing derivatives are morphine and heroine. They both, like majority of dependency producing opioids, bind to opioid receptors.

Acute intoxication

This is characterized by apathy, bradycardia, hypotension, respiratory depression subnormal core body temperature and pinpoint pupils. In severe intoxication, mydriasis may occur due to hypoxia.

Withdrawal syndrome

The onset of withdrawal symptoms occurs typically within 12-24 hours, has a peak within 24-72 hours and symptoms subside within 7-10 days of the last dose of opioid. The characteristic symptoms include lacrimation, rhinorrhoea, papillary dilation, sweating, diarrhoea, tachycardia, mild hypertension, insomnia, raised body temperature, muscle cramps, body ache, severe anxiety, nausea, vomiting and anorexia. The heroine withdrawal syndrome is more severe than the withdrawal syndrome of morphine.

Treatment

Before treatment, a correct diagnosis must be made on the basis of history, examination and laboratory tests. These tests are:

1) Naloxone challenge test9 to precipitate the withdrawal symptoms).
2) Urinary opioids testing: with radio immune assay (RIA), free radical assay technique, thin layer chromatography,

high pressure liquid chromatography or enzyme multiplied immune-assay technique.

The treatment can be divided into 3 main types:

❖ Treatment of overdose
❖ Detoxification
❖ Maintenance therapy

CANNABIS USE DISORDER

Cannabis is derived from the hemp plant, cannabis sativa, which has several varieties named after the region in which it is found. cannabis produces a very mild physical dependence, with a relatively mild withdrawal syndrome characterised by fine tremors, irritability, restlessness, nervousness, insomnia, decreased appetite and craving. The syndrome begins within few hours of stopping cannabis use and lasts for 4-5 days.

Acute intoxication

Mild cannabis intoxication is characterised by mild impairment of consciousness and orientation, light headedness, tachycardia, a sense of floating in the air, a euphoric dream- like state, alternation in psychomotor activities and tremors in addition to photophobia, lacrimation, tachycardia, reddening of conjunctiva, dry mouth and increased appetite. Perceptual disturbances are common and include depersonalization, derealisation, synaesthesia (sensation in one sensory modality caused by a sensation in another sensory modality, eg. Seeing the music) and increased sensitivity to sound.

Complications

The complications of cannabis use include :

a) Transient or short lasting psychiatric disorders: acute anxiety, paranoid psychosis, hysterical fugue- like states, suicidal ideation, hypomania, schizophrenia like state, acute organic psychosis and very rarely, depression.

b) A motivational syndrome: chronic cannabis use is postulated to cause lethargy, apathy, loss of interest, reduced drive and lack of ambition.

c) Hemp insanity or cannabis psychosis it was described as being similar to acute schizophreniform disorder with disorientation and confusion, and with a good prognosis.

Other complications:

memory impairment, worsening or relapse in schizophrenia or mood disorder, chronic obstructive airway disease, pulmonary malignancy and increased risk for the developing foetus if taken during pregnancy

COCAINE USE DISORDER

Cocaine is an alkaloid derived from the coca bush, Erythroxylum coca, found in Bolivia and Peru. Cocaine is a central stimulant which inhibits the reuptake of dopamine along with that of norepinephrine and serotonin.

Acute intoxication

Acute cocaine intoxication is characterised by papillary dilatation, tachycardia, hypertension, sweating, and nausea or vomiting. Later judgement is impaired and there is impairment of social and occupational functioning.

Withdrawal symptoms

Cocaine use produces a very mild physical, but a very strong psychic, dependence.

Complications

The complications of chronic cocaine use include acute anxiety reaction, uncontrolled compulsive behaviour, psychotic episodes, delirium and delusional disorders. High doses of cocaine can induce seizures, respiratory depression, cardiac arrhythmias, coronary artery occlusion, myocardial infarction, lung damage and gastrointestinal necrosis.

Treatment

Treatment of cocaine overdose

The treatment consists of oxygenation, muscle relaxants, and IV thiopentone and/or IV diazepam (for seizures and severe anxiety). IV propranolol, a specific antagonist of cocaine induced sympathomimetic effects, can be used in a dose of 1mg every minute.

Treatment of chronic cocaine use

The treatment of underlying or co-existent psychopathology is the most important step in the management of chronic cocaine use. The pharmacological treatment include the use of bromocriptine(a dopaminergic agonist) and amantadine (an antiparkinsonian) in reducing cocaine craving. Other useful drugs are Desipramine, imipramine and trazodone(both for reducing craving and for antidepressant effect). The goal of treatment is total abstinence from cocaine use.

AMPHETAMINE USE DISORDER

Amphetamine refers to a unique chemical which is precisely phenyl-iso-propylamine or methyl-phenethyl-amine. It is a powerful CNS stimulant, with peripheral sympathomimetic effects. Although still clinically indicated for narcolepsy, attention deficit hyperactivity disorder, one of the commonest patterns of use is seen among students and sports persons to overcome the need for sleep and fatigue. Tolerance usually develops to the central as well as cardiovascular effects of amphetamine.

Intoxication and complication

The signs and symptoms of acute amphetamine intoxication are primarily cardiovascular (tachycardia, hypertension, haemorrhage, cardiac failure and cardiovascular shock) and central (seizures, hyperpyrexia, tremors, ataxia, euphoria, papillary dilatation and coma). The neuropsychiatric manifestations include anxiety, panic, insomnia, restlessness, irritability and hostility).

Acute intoxication may present as a paranoid hallucinatory syndrome which closely mimics paranoid schizophrenia. However a confident diagnosis requires estimation of urinary amphetamine level. Chronic amphetamine intoxication leads to severe, compulsive craving for the drug. A high degree of tolerance is characteristic, with the dependent individual needing up to 15-20 times the initial dose in order to obtain the pleasurable effects. Tactile hallucination in clear consciousness, may sometimes occur in chronic amphetamine intoxication.

Withdrawal syndrome

The withdrawal syndrome is typically seen on abrupt discontinuation of amphetamine after a period of chronic use. It is characterised by depression, marked asthenia, apathy, fatigue agitation and hyperplasia.

Treatment

Acute intoxication is treated by symptomatic measures, eg. Hyperpyrexia (cold sponging, parenteral antipyretics), seizures (parentraldiazepams), psychotic symptoms(haloperidol), and hypertension (antihypertensive).Treatment of withdrawal symptoms include antidepressants and supportive psychotherapy

LSD use disorders

Lysergic acid diethylamide, first synthesised by Albert Hoffman in 1938 and popularly known as 'acid', is a powerful hallucinogen. LSD presumably produces its effects by an action on the 5-HT levels in brain. Although tolerance and psychological dependence occur with LCD use, no physical dependence or withdrawal syndrome is reported.

Intoxication

The characteristic features of acute LCD intoxication are perceptual changes occurring in clear consciousness and autonomic hyperactivity. These changes are usually associated with marked anxiety or depression, thought euphoria is more common in small doses. Sometimes, acute LCD intoxication presents with an acute panic reaction, known as a bad trip, in which the individual experiences a loss of control over his self. The recovery usually occurs within 8-12 hours of the last dose. No withdrawal symptoms have been described with LSD use. The complications of chronic LCD use include psychiatric symptoms and occasionally foetal abnormalities.

Treatment

The treatment of acute LCD intoxication consists of symptomatic management with antianxiety, antidepressants or antipsychotic medication along with supportive psychotherapy

Barbiturate use disorders

Barbiturate use disorders are now subsumed under the sedative, hypnotic and anxiolytic use disorders. The commonly abused barbiturates are secobarbital, pentobarbital produce marked physical and psychological dependence. Tolerance (both central and metabolic) develops rapidly and is usually marked. There is also a cross tolerance with alcohol.

Intoxication and complication

Acute intoxication, typically occurring as an episodic phenomenon, is characterised by irritability, increased productivity of speech, incoordination, attention and memory impairment, and ataxia. Intravenous use can lead to skin abscesses, cellulitis, embolism and hypersensitivity reaction

Withdrawal reaction

The barbiturate withdrawal syndrome can be very severe. It usually occurs in individuals who are taking more than 600-800 mg/day of secobarbital equivalent for more than one month. It is characterised by marked restlessness, tremors, hypertension, seizures, a psychosis resembling delirium termers. The withdrawal syndrome is at its worst about 72 hours after the last dose. Coma, followed by death, can occur in some cases.

TREATMENT

The barbiturate intoxication should be treated symptomatically. If the patient is conscious, induction of vomiting and use of activated charcoal can reduce the absorption. If coma ensues, intensive care measures should be employed on emergency basis. Phenobarbital substitution therapy has been suggested for the treatment of withdrawal from short acting barbiturates. After the detoxification phase is over, follow-up supportive treatment and treatment of associated psychiatric disorder, usually depression, are important to prevent relapses.

Benzodiazepines and other sedative-hypnotic use disorder

Since the discovery of chlordiazepines in 1957 by Sternbach, benzodiazepines have replaced other sedative-hypnotics in the treatment of insomnia and anxiety. These are currently one of the most often prescribed drugs. Benzodiazepines produce their effects by acting on benzodiazepine receptors (GABA-benzodiazepine receptor complex), thereby indirectly increasing the action of GABA).

REFERENCES:

- Niraj Ahuja - A short text book of psychiatry 5th edition. Jay Pee -2002.
- S. Nambi: Psychiatry for Nurses, first edition Jay Pee Company – 1998,
- Bimla Kapoor   - "Text Book Of Psychiatric Nursing" 1st edition – volume II, Delhi-1994.
- Lynda Juall Carpentio- "Handbook of Nursing Diagnosis. 7th edition- Lipincott – New York 1997.
- Elakkuvanabhaskars's "text book of nursing education", 2nd edition, EMMESS, medical publishers, page no -192-194.
- R.sudha "Nursing education" jaypee publication 2013,page no:40
- KP 'Neeraja' The text book of essentials of mental health nursing, jaypee brothers medical publication, page no; 570-589.
- Gail w.stuart, michele t.laraia" principles and practice of psychiatry nursing' 8th edition, publisher by Elsevier, page no; 220
- Mary c. townsand, text book of mental health nursing & psychiatric nursing, jaypee publishers, page no: 845-851.
- Damson SJ, Sellman JD. Five-year outcomes of alcohol-dependent persons treated with motivational enhancement. Journal of Studies on Alcohol and Drugs. 2008;69:589–593.

Printed in Great Britain
by Amazon

48566639R00036